Spark!

Weight Loss Coaching Questions

Jill Brook, Nutritionist

Why & How?

Why I Wrote This

I wanted to share a simple way to spark more success. Whether you are coaching clients professionally or helping a loved one informally, or even just coaching yourself, a simple change of approach can make all the difference! It's easy, and makes the weight loss process so much more interesting and enjoyable...*and effective!*

Why is Weight Coaching So Tricky?

Weight loss coaching isn't like other types of coaching!

For one thing, most people already *know* what they should do to slim down. Television, books and media have already educated them on the main *shoulds* of healthy weight loss. If they *could* simply eat less, exercise more, and replace processed foods with veggies, then they *would have succeeded already!* Clients can feel insulted when their coach doesn't acknowledge this.

Secondly, no tennis coach, speech coach, writing coach, or business coach asks so much of her clients. A weight loss coach asks her clients to alter their biology, daily routines, habits, lifestyle, social interactions, reward structures, and even brain chemistry. These are some of the most sacred parts of a person's life! They are unique, complex and only their owner can begin to know them completely enough to manipulate them responsibly.

What's more, any well-intentioned coaching advice risks triggering the rebellious voices, those inner thoughts that say things like:

- "You don't understand me."
- "That would never work for me."
- "I tried that already. Do you think I'm an idiot?"
- "I tried that and failed. I'm pathetic."
- "I know that already. This is insulting."
- "I hate this. I should just read a book on this instead."

That's obviously not helpful!

So how does a weight loss coach guide a client to lasting success? In my experience, there's one and only one way: **By asking the right questions.**

Let me be more specific: By **never** telling a client what do to. By **only** asking the client questions that spark progress on her own terms. This is not to say that a coach never conveys information, or guides with a strong hand, but that she strategically does it within smart questions.

This leads the client to engage more deeply, and to come up with her *own* best solutions, which are the *only* ones likely to stick and succeed.

Why Questions?

Over 15 years of nutrition

coaching, I have learned time and again that asking the *right questions* is almost always the best tool for helping clients make progress each day. Whether a client is just getting started, progressing smoothly, feeling "stuck," or struggling with any number of challenges, I find that **questions consistently work.**

Why? Because a good question leads a client to:

- Feel more deeply **engaged and empowered**
- Take **ownership** for her actions and choices
- Get comfortable with her own **personal idiosyncrasies**
- Examine the hidden **costs and benefits** of her choices
- Make the **smartest compromises** when she has conflicting needs or desires
- Devise and test **creative solutions**

- Have **epiphanies and breakthroughs**, and perhaps most importantly
- Come up with her **own best lifestyles** for overall health and happiness

A coach's best lecturing, advising, cheerleading, scolding, or critiquing can't do these. Questions can!

Let's take an example, where a coach might be tempted to state something like "Granola bars aren't healthy - you should eat an apple instead." Look out! The client's inner rebellious voices may be stirring to life, perhaps with angry retorts, like "I know but..." or "I hate apples" or "I'm going to scream if I have to give up one more tasty treat" or any number of other unproductive responses. Instead, the coach could ask "Can you think of some less processed options, ones that will get you better results, but still be satisfying to you?" The question engages instead of insults, and initiates productive problem-solving.

I've trained dozens of coaches and even the most brilliant, insightful and charismatic ones get better results when they adopt this one rule: **Always ask. Never tell.**

Questions Make Good Coaches Great

A good coach might appear simply to be having a pleasant conversation, but she is actually working hard to:

- Keep a client focused on implementing practical solutions, rather than thinking "I just need to try harder."

- Act as a sounding board, to

help clients work out their ideas, emotions and plans.

- Help turn negative emotions, like frustration, into productive energy and a specific game plan.

- Probe for details, because a plan isn't likely to succeed unless the specifics are worked out. Plus, mentally rehearsing a plan makes it robust.

- Make sure a client considers all options - along with the consequences - before choosing one.

- Make sure clients keep their own best long-term interests in mind. The allure of fast weight loss - at the cost of metabolism or lean tissue - is a common threat that coaches guard against.

- Prompt clients to resolve inconsistencies that come from competing needs, such as juggling family, career, finances, social life, etc., in addition to wellness goals. This often means probing about priorities, what is realistic, or what promotes best all-around happiness, rather than just best fitness.

- Provide accountability and focus, so that a client's demanding life doesn't steal away too much attention from health goals.

- Help prioritize daily or weekly to-do items, keeping them appropriately ambitious but manageable.

- Lend positive energy to help a client learn and rebound from inevitable low points.

- Make the weight loss process more enjoyable, by providing support, empathy and maybe even a sense of humor about all of the grueling work involved.

- Generally keep clients motivated, on-track and working *smart* toward their goals.

Good coaches do all of those things and more. The very best coaches I've seen, however, do all of those things in a special way: **With questions!**

How Do I Craft the Right Question?

First, *listen!* You cannot possibly choose a good question if you are doing all the talking! The right question depends on where the client is at the exact moment. Is she frustrated? Motivated? Prepared? Focused? Feeling deprived? Stuck? The right question is the one that helps the client make progress from their current state, whatever that happens to be...which you can only know by listening closely.

Second, *practice!* Whenever I talk to an inexperienced coach about asking questions, the response I get is typically something like: "That's impossible. How can I help a client if I can't *tell* her anything?"

My response: Try it! Practice via role play and force yourself *never* to tell, *always* to ask. I think you'll be surprised at how much *more* powerful your coaching can be.

And finally, *adapt!* The questions in this book are grouped into common scenarios that arise frequently. Perhaps these will suit your needs, but are intended to be a jumping off point. In most cases, you'll want to build your own questions, drawing upon various parts of this book, your own experiences, your communication style, the attributes of your client, and so on. Your exact choice of words, voice intonation, facial expression, body language and timing can all make a difference. A fun challenge of coaching is adapting the questions and their delivery style to fit each client's unique needs and personality.

How Can I Best Use Questions?

In my experience, clients make the most progress when they are prompted to:

- Contemplate 1-3 big questions per day.

- Be exhaustive, because it forces them to think of *all* possible solutions, even the unconventional.

- Answer in detail. Explaining a game plan in detail serves as the mental run-through that promotes success.

- Speak aloud or write down answers, because the extra accountability makes a huge difference.

- Answer only the questions most relevant to the current situation. The chapters help guide you.

- Answer honestly, without fear of judgment. This should be an interesting opportunity for a client to get to know herself, to embrace her unique needs, quirks and idiosyncrasies and to use this knowledge to brainstorm creative solutions.

- Consider which tradeoffs and compromises would make her *happiest* (not only fittest) in the long run.

The questions in this book are designed to help a client feel happier, healthier, wiser and closer to her goal, no matter where she is in her journey.

Good luck using the art of questions, and may you enjoy the thrill of sparking much success!

All my best,

Jill Brook

CHAPTER 1

Got the
Winning
Mindset?

In my experience, the most
successful clients have a few things
in common. They have:

- *Intrinsic* motivation, rather
  than wanting just to please
  others, such as a concerned
  doctor or spouse
- Realistic expectations for what
  results are achievable, and

how much effort will be required
- Readiness to make permanent changes
- Interest in the process itself, rather than only the final result.

These questions are designed to help clients get the winning mindset.

What are your goals?

For example:

- *Reach a goal weight?*
- *Gain _ pounds of muscle?*
- *Lose _ inches in the waist?*
- *Stop craving sugar?*
- *Change a specific habit?*

When was the last time you reached each of these goals, if ever?

Are your goals realistic for your body, genetics and age?

Are they realistic for your lifestyle, and the amount of time and energy you plan to expend?

Can you choose a goal *range*, rather than a single number?

For example:

- *Lose ½ to 2 pounds per week?*
- *Maintain a body fat percent between 20 and 25%?*

Why do you want to change your eating habits?

What benefits will you reap in the long term? In the short term?

What daily behaviors will be necessary to reach your goal?

Which of these will be enjoyable and which will be difficult?

Which temporary discomforts are you willing to endure?

For example:

- *Cravings?*
- *Hunger?*
- *Feeling deprived?*

Are you prepared for some temporary blandness until your taste buds change?

Have you experienced changing taste buds before?

Are you prepared to embrace inevitable failures as valuable learning experiences?

How will you keep yourself from becoming discouraged?

How will you use mistakes to get smarter and more successful, rather than discouraged?

Would it help to keep a "lessons learned" journal?

Are you ready to lose fat slowly, to avoid losing muscle and lowering your metabolism?

How will you resist any temptation to "crash diet"?

Which habits are you willing to change for life, and not just temporarily?

Which are you *not* willing to change permanently?

Are you open to doing some self-experiments, to find what works best for you?

Have you tried this in the past and learned anything valuable?

Which of your personality traits will make this easier?

For example:

- *Being organized?*
- *Being a good planner?*
- *Enjoying cooking?*

How can you put these to good use?

Which of your personality traits will make this harder?

For example:

- *Being a perfectionist?*
- *Being known as the life of the party?*
- *Hating routines?*

How can you keep these traits from derailing your progress?

Does a weight program feel exciting and interesting or more like oppressive drudgery?

How can you make the necessary daily work more interesting, fun or bearable?

Have you ever tried to change any major habits in the past?

For example:

- *Quitting smoking?*
- *Taking up exercise?*
- *Giving up alcohol?*

What was that like? Did it teach you anything?

Have you ever trained a new behavior in a child or puppy?

How much did consistency, routine and repetition make a difference? Ready to train your brain in a similar fashion?

What are your biggest challenges to healthier eating?

For example:

- *No time to prepare?*
- *Busy social life?*
- *In love with eating?*

What in your life makes it easier to eat right?

How will you replace the lost pleasure when you give up some tasty treats?

What will you do - besides eat - when your brain cries out for pleasure?

CHAPTER 2

Have your
Best Eating
Plan?

Successful clients figure out
exactly what foods work best for
them, in terms of taste,
satisfaction, convenience, cost,
dietary restrictions, and so on.
This is not only valuable for
cementing healthy routines, but
also defends against that all-too-
common situation where a client

hears conflicting advice about what to eat, feels confused, and finally says "scr*w it, I'll have the cheesecake!"

Which foods make you feel most satisfied?

Which matters more to you - feeling physically satisfied or emotionally satisfied from your food?

What healthy foods are enjoyable to you?

Got something from every food group - fruits, veggies, proteins, whole grains, dairy, nuts, seeds, beans, legumes, herbs, spices?

What vegetables do you like?

Prepared how?

Because vegetables are crucial to success, what additional veggies are you willing to try?

What veggies are worth trying again after your taste buds have a chance to change?

What are your "Teaser Foods," which stimulate more hunger, rather than satisfy?

When is it worth it to eat a Teaser Food?

Do you need to learn some new food skills?

For example:

- *Making a good stir-fry?*
- *Using a grill?*
- *Following a recipe?*

How and when will you learn?

What will be your Go-To Snacks?

Which snacks should you leave in your office, car, purse, briefcase, etc., in case of emergency?

What will be your Go-To Breakfasts?

What breakfasts will you enjoy on weekends, at restaurants, or when you have more time?

What will be your Go-To Lunches?

What will you order when at restaurants? How can you get more veggies into your lunches?

What will be your Go-To Dinners?

What will you order when at restaurants? How can you get more "clean" veggies into your dinners?

What are your "emergency dinner" plans, for when you need a quick healthy dinner?

What "emergency dinner" items do you need to keep stocked in your kitchen?

What are your Go-To beverages?

What calorie-free beverages are most exciting and satisfying to you? What will you order at a cafe or a bar?

What are your healthy Go-To restaurants?

What should you order there?

When eating out, what will you look for on the menu?

Are you willing to make special requests, like getting sauces on the side or ordering off-menu?

CHAPTER 3

Starting

Strong?

Especially when a client is just starting out, it's valuable to check in frequently - perhaps daily - to see that she is working *smart*, feeling good and seeing results. Any problems should be corrected as early as possible. Good coaches help clients to anticipate challenges, stay prepared and remain detail-oriented, so that the smart daily behaviors can most quickly turn into automatic habits.

Great results right from the start can also boost commitment and motivation. These questions help promote a strong start.

What did you eat in the past 24 hours?

Is there anything you wish you had done differently?

Did your choices feel "worth it"?

If not, what would you do differently next time you are in the same situation?

What are your eating plans for the next 24 hours?

What about the next 48 hours?

In the coming week, do you expect any big challenges to your healthy eating?

What is your game plan for navigating those challenges?

How many hours of good sleep did you get last night?

If you are sleep-deprived, can you make time to catch up before it causes cravings, hunger and will power problems?

Feeling prepared for the next 24-48 hours?

If not, what do you need to do to get prepared?

CHAPTER 4

Progressing
Smoothly?

When a client is losing weight and feeling great, it's tempting for a coach to simply cheer, high-five and enjoy the success. But good coaches don't do that! Instead, they help the client figure out *why* things are going so well, and then *document* those findings in case the client gets off track later. Knowing how she was eating, thinking and managing her time may be valuable to get back on track.

These questions help to elucidate keys to success, and to foresee and protect against challenges that could throw the client off-track.

What are your Go-To meals and snacks?

Because documenting exactly what works is extremely valuable, can you be any more specific?

What exercise routine is working for you?

What other details can you document, about when, where, how long, how intense, with whom...?

What is your current grocery shopping and food prep routine?

Specifically when, where and how do you complete the prep work that is getting you success?

Who is helping you succeed?

For example:

- *Spouse?*
- *Friends?*
- *Coworkers?*
- *Personal trainer?*
- *Paid helper?*
- *Weight coach?*

Who makes it easier to eat right and how do they help?

What time are you getting to bed and waking up?

What helps you sleep well?

How are you managing stress?

For example:

- *Exercise?*
- *Meditation?*
- *Just lucky; stress is naturally low right now?*

How can you prevent unnecessary stress from arising?

What could get you off track?

What can you do to help prevent that?

What advice would your current "On Track Self" give to yourself in the future if you fell off track?

What should you remember or do first, in the event that you get off track?

CHAPTER 5

Recently

Indulge?

After "blowing it," a client is likely to feel frustrated, ashamed or even like giving up. A good coach can redirect that negative energy into valuable learning and productive action, so that the client feels wiser and better for the experience, ready to rebound like a champ!

These questions get you started.

Was it worth it?

Was there considerable joy, fun, social bonding, good memories attached to the splurge?

Did it have delayed or hidden costs?

For example:

- *Rebound hunger?*
- *Stretched stomach?*
- *Blitzed taste buds?*
- *Cravings triggered?*
- *Sleep made fitful?*
- *Old addiction awakened?*

Does this change the "worth it" calculation?

What would you do differently next time?

For example:

- *Bring snacks with you?*
- *Give away the party leftovers?*
- *Give a donation, rather than buying Girl Scout cookies?*

What was the trigger?

For example:

- *A particular person?*
- *An emotion?*
- *A physical location?*

How can you avoid being vulnerable to this trigger again?

What lessons did it teach you?

Assuming you can't change your will power, what can you do to implement the lessons learned?

What can you do *right now* that will help you do better next time?

How does this help you avoid your triggers or minimize their impact next time?

Do you want to make this "failure" a turning point?

How can you rebound from a "failure" in such a way that is so valuable that you are glad it happened?

CHAPTER 6

Struggling with
Motivation?

Coaches can boost motivation by helping clients:

- Focus on their *intrinsic* motivators
- Focus only on their next 1-3 specific steps
- Break down intimidating tasks into smaller sub-tasks, until they feel manageable
- Feel optimally challenged
- Focus on executing important

daily behaviors, rather than on the ultimate result, which is proven to impede success
- Helping clients avoid motivation-killers, like stress and sleep deprivation.

These questions help you get started.

What is in this for *you*?

For example:

- *Better sleep?*
- *Improved energy?*
- *Less pain?*

How many *selfish* reasons can you find to improve your habits?

What's the *short-term* pay-off to eating healthy today?

For example:

- *Feeling great?*
- *Sleeping better?*
- *Having better digestion?*

How many different *immediate* positives are there?

What healthy acts can you do today, no matter how small?

For example:

- *Drink 8 cups water?*
- *Walk?*
- *Plan tomorrow's meals?*

Can some of these things be turned into regular habits?

Are you tired, overworked, overwhelmed, sleep-deprived, in pain, or stressed right now?

How can you address this?

Do you have the *time* to grocery shop and prepare healthy food in a relaxed, non-hurried way?

How will you make time for this?

Who inspires you and why?

How can you spend more time with them?

Which friends can you recruit for support?

What exactly should you say to gain their support?

Would a friendly bet or challenge help keep you on track?

For example:

- *Anyone at work caught drinking soda owes $10?*

What are the specifics of a bet that sounds motivating?

Are you intimidated by how distant your goal feels?

What is a smaller initial goal that feels reachable?

Are you focusing too much on your final goal, rather than the daily behaviors that will achieve it?

What healthy things *can* you do every day or week?

What 3 daily behaviors should you prioritize?

For example:

- *Getting to the grocery store?*
- *Getting to bed by 10pm?*
- *Eating a salad at lunch?*

Can you commit to these for a week and see if they start to get easy and automatic?

What time of day are you most energized and productive?

Can you plan, organize and prepare your food at this time?

CHAPTER 7

Struggling with
Cravings?

A good coach can guide a client to understand and prevent most cravings...and then have a good game plan for when resistance is futile. These questions get you started.

How does it feel to have a craving?

Next time you are craving, can you observe it and acknowledge it, without immediately assuming it must be fed?

Could there be a physical cause?

For example:

- *Dehydration?*
- *Need quick energy?*
- *Exhaustion?*
- *Salt depletion after heavy sweating?*

How can you prevent or address these problems in a healthy way?

What might help distract you for 10 minutes?

For example:

- *Calling a friend?*
- *Taking a shower?*
- *Checking email?*

Where can you keep this list, so that it's easy to review when a craving hits?

What healthy food would "inoculate" you?

For example:

- *Tomatoes, basil and string cheese to prevent pizza craving?*
- *Baked apples to prevent apple pie craving?*
- *Cocoa nibs to prevent chocolate craving?*

When you crave, what is your brain really seeking?

For example:

- *Comfort?*
- *Pain relief?*
- *Entertainment?*
- *Energy?*

What are healthier ways to satisfy these needs?

Which foods seem to trigger new cravings?

Should you give up these foods entirely and find substitutes that don't trigger cravings?

Is Taste Bud Ping Pong at play?

Should you experiment with avoiding that first strong flavor (sweet, salty or bitter), to see if you have fewer cravings all day?

If Taste Bud Ping Pong is a factor, what is the trigger?

For example:

- *Hidden sweet flavors, like in many toothpastes?*
- *Splenda, stevia, or other noncaloric sweeteners?*
- *Healthful but salty foods, like tuna, cottage cheese, pickles?*
- *Strong bitter coffee or tea?*

For cravings that must be indulged, what are the healthiest foods that will satisfy?

What specific ingredients should you have on hand?

If you crave sweets, what are some relatively healthy foods that satisfy?

What other healthy-ish foods will satisfy other cravings, such as salty, crunchy, fatty or other cravings?

CHAPTER 8

Struggling with
Self
Control?

Many clients blame themselves for bad will power and resolve repeatedly to "try harder next time." If that was a good approach, it would have worked by now! There is a better solution.

A good coach can help clients identify and manage the specific *controllable* factors that strengthen their self-control.

These questions get you started.

Is there a time of day that is hardest for you?

What pleasant activity can you schedule for that time, to keep you busily engaged?

What locations or environments are toughest for you?

How can you minimize your time there?

Does sleep make a big difference?

How can you stay better rested?

What tricks or strategies seem to help?

For example:

- *Chewing gum?*
- *Brushing and flossing right after dinner?*
- *Keeping temptations out of the house?*

What other strategies should you try experimentally?

Which specific foods make you lose self control?

Which foods are easier to avoid entirely, rather than trying to eat in moderation?

Which foods should be banned from your home?

If your family refuses to ban some of these, where could they hide them out of your sight?

What mantra should you think of when temptation strikes?

For example:

- *"I refuse to let food own me!"*

Would it help to write it out and tape it to your fridge?

Whom can you tell about your goals, for accountability?

How else could they be asked to help keep you in line? With friendly bets? By promising not to tempt you? By removing temptations from your field of view or home?

How does it feel to exert self control, rather than to "cave in?"

When is the last time you overcame the urge to overeat? What did that feel like? Can you think about that feeling next time you are tempted?

CHAPTER 9

Struggling with
Convenience?

Convenience is a powerful force! A good coach can help clients find time-saving short-cuts and strategies. They can also help clients realize the utmost importance of preparation - versus "winging it" - and prompt them to carve out time for weekly prep routines that can quickly become automatic habits. These questions get you started.

When could you incorporate a weekly prep session, to get lots of meals and snacks ready?

If you can't get the entire week prepared, what is your plan for the remaining meals?

Who could help prepare healthy foods for you and how?

For example:

- *Could you give a weekly grocery list to your spouse, assistant or neighbor?*

Can you write down your specific food needs for any helpers, so that they are guaranteed to prepare the right things?

What "emergency meals" should you put in your pantry and freezer?

How often should you restock these? Can you put it on your calendar right now?

What foods should you bring to work every Monday, to last the entire week?

For example:

- *5 Greek yogurts*
- *Package of low fat string cheese*
- *Bag of apples*

Can you put a reminder in your schedule right now?

Which Emergency Snacks should you keep in your car, purse, desk drawer, etc?

For example:

- *1oz bags of almonds?*
- *Wasa crackers?*

Can you schedule a weekly time to refill these stashes?

Do you need to buy a small cooler, lunch box, thermos, or good containers to carry food with you?

Specifically, what should you get?

Which gadgets or appliances would save you time?

For example:

- *George Foreman Grill?*
- *Crock Pot?*
- *Mini-fridge for the office?*

What should you buy, borrow or set out, so that it's ready to use?

Should you look into meal delivery services?

For example:

- *Local restaurants that deliver?*
- *Meal delivery services, like ZEN Foods?*

If this is too expensive to do long-term, then what is your plan for afterward?

To simplify preparation, which meals can you repeat weekly?

Specifically, which meals will happen which days?

To simplify grocery shopping, what foods should you buy every single time?

Can you put a list on your smart phone, so that you always have it handy?

Which take-out meals or restaurant entrees are healthy and convenient enough to use often?

Should you add their phone numbers to your cell phone, for easy ordering?

CHAPTER 10

Struggling with a
Plateau?

The coach's first task is to figure out whether the client is truly at a plateau, or whether their results are acceptably slow. I like to remind my clients that even a quarter pound of fat equals a stick of butter removed from the body. Slow results are more maintainable, less likely to slow the metabolism, and require less deprivation. I'm a fan of slow, steady results. That said, if a client is working hard and not seeing results, it's time to figure out why! These questions get you started.

Are you truly plateaued or just losing weight slowly?

Would you be happy with this pace of weight loss by the end of a year?

Could you be gaining weight from muscle, which boosts strength and metabolism?

Should you schedule a body composition test?

Has impatience caused you to fail in the past?

How can you remind yourself to be more patient?

Are there times when you are eating more than you need to?

When could you eat less without going hungry or weak?

Which 500 calories per week offer you the least nutrition and pleasure?

Want to try cutting out those calories and see what happens?

Should you have your thyroid or hormones checked by a doctor?

What does your doctor suggest to break your weight plateau?

Are you exercising too much, too little or ineffectively?

Should you consult a fitness expert?

Are you sleep deprived or exhausted or extremely stressed?

What can you do to change or manage these things?

Want to try turning down your thermostat, to boost metabolism?

How about making your beverages very icy?

Are you deluding yourself about the quantities you eat?

Should you measure everything you eat for three days?

Could your restaurant meals be worse than you thought?

Can you avoid eating at restaurants for a week to find out?

What food or exercise habits are you willing to change to see better results?

Want to try it for two weeks, to see if it helps?

Using your smart phone, can you photograph everything you eat for a week?

Do your photos show any obvious ways you could improve?

CHAPTER 11

Struggling with
Hunger?

The first thing to do with a hungry client is to make sure she isn't under-eating! Hunger with faster weight loss might be a sign that she needs to eat more, or else risk losing lean tissue and metabolism.

If under-eating isn't a problem, then the coach can help guide the client to assess whether sleep deprivation, stress, poor food choices, eating too fast or dehydration might be the cause. Good coaches can also lead clients to find dietary changes that help clients feel more satisfied without gaining weight, such as choosing higher-satiety foods, chewing more times per bite and eating more slowly.

These questions get you started.

How does true hunger feel for you?

How does does it feel different from cravings, thirst, desire to eat out of boredom, etc.?

Are you eating enough protein?

Should you try eating a higher protein breakfast?

Are you eating enough fiber?

Should you try getting more fiber at breakfast?

Which foods stimulate your appetite, rather than satisfy it?

What satisfying replacements can you find for these foods?

How much do sleep and stress affect your appetite?

Could you experiment with earlier bedtimes for one week?

Are you getting enough sound sleep?

Can you designate one night per week (or month) to get *completely* caught up on sleep?

Could you replace any of your regular foods with more filling choices?

For example:

- *Peanuts instead of peanut butter?*
- *Corn on the cob instead of corn tortillas?*
- *Fresh fruit instead of smoothies?*

How quickly do you eat compared to others?

Do you always sit down and relax to eat?

Could you eat more slowly?

What tricks should you use to slow yourself down?

Could you cut your food into smaller pieces?

How will you remember to do this?

Could you chew each bite 35+ times before swallowing?

How will you remind yourself to do this?

Are you drinking enough water?

Does your hunger go away when you drink water?

Could you eat more of your food earlier in the day?

What preparation will help you eat more at breakfast or early snack times, to prevent hunger later?

CHAPTER 12

Struggling with

Food- Boredom?

Fixing food-boredom can often be as simple as helping the client think of new foods, cooking methods, combinations, flavorings or textures to try.

Other times, food-boredom can signal a general malaise. Clients may be looking to food for excitement or novelty when really it's *other* parts of their lives lacking pizzazz.

Either way, these questions guide a client to discover their best solutions.

Want to explore more ethnic foods?

What places and flavors sound interesting to you?

Can you spice up old favorites with ethnic flavorings?

For example:

- *Chicken with Indian spices?*
- *Fish with molé sauce?*
- *African spiced veggies?*

When can you make time to do a little research or experiment with spice combinations?

What novel food have you always been curious to eat?

How can you use it to make something reasonably healthy?

Where could you find some novel healthy ideas?

For example:

- *Cooking magazines?*
- *Menus or cookbooks from famous spas?*
- *Websites?*
- *Whole Foods Market prepared foods section?*

When will you carve out time for this?

What rare foods have you never tried?

For example:

- *Dragon fruit?*
- *Quail eggs?*
- *Saffron?*
- *Elk?*
- *Black forbidden rice?*

When and where can you shop for these?

What is new and exciting in your life right now?

Besides yummy foods, what do you look forward to enjoying in the near future?

Is it possible that you are bored with other aspects of your life and asking food to fill the void?

If so, what could you do for stimulation besides eat?

What are some *non*-edible delights in your life?

How can you get more of them? Which can you schedule *right now*?

CHAPTER 13

Struggling with an
Urge to
Splurge?

A growing desire to splurge can be a desire for pleasure, stimulation, an energy boost, an addictive "hit," a rebellion against dietary rules, or many other things. A good coach can help a client figure out what her brain or body *really* wants, and then find the healthiest way to satisfy that need.

These questions get you started.

What kind of splurge are you wanting?

What triggered the desire?

What would be the price of giving in?

For example:

- *Weight gain?*
- *Feeling ill?*
- *Triggering cravings?*
- *Awakening addiction?*

Would your long-term happiness be higher if you give in?

Is this splurge a means to feeling a particular way?

For example:

- *Feeling energized?*
- *Boosting mood?*
- *Feeling comforted?*
- *Feeling indulged?*

How else could you get this same feeling?

Imagine you just gave in: How do you feel?

Imagine it's a day or week after the splurge: Now how do you feel?

What *non-edible* indulgences do you enjoy?

For example:

- *Bubble baths?*
- *Shopping?*
- *Reading?*
- *Sleeping in?*

Would any of these satisfy your need?

How can you reward yourself in a healthier way?

What is the healthiest food that would satisfy your desire to splurge?

If you plan to splurge, can you do it early in the day?

Can you "sandwich" it between healthy meals, like salad or other veggies?

CHAPTER 14

Struggling with
Social
Situations?

Social settings are no problem for some clients, while others find them torturously full of temptation, pressure and awkwardness. A good coach can help a struggling client to:

- Decide how much she is willing to be different from the crowd

- Strategize a smart game plan for specific situations

- Practice phrases that make it easier to decline edible offerings

- Recruit helpers to offer emotional support, accountability or even practical help.

These questions get you started.

Which social situations are toughest for you?

What specifically makes it tough - the edible temptations or the social pressure to fit in?

When is it worth it to eat or drink out of social obligation?

What are the pros and cons of eating poorly to fit in?

Which friends or family are good influences on your eating habits?

How can you spend more time with these people?

Which friends or family are bad influences on your habits?

How can you make them exert less bad influence?

What phrases can help you gracefully decline offered food?

For example:

- *"No thanks, but it smells wonderful!"*
- *"It pains me to decline, but I must."*

Do you need to practice your phrases aloud, so they will come more naturally?

What phrases can help you gracefully decline alcoholic beverages?

Do you need to practice reciting these aloud several times, to help them come more naturally?

Whose support would help you eat better?

What can you say to them to bring them "on board" and make them supportive?

What are some fun social activities that don't involve overeating?

For example:

- *Hiking?*
- *Board games?*
- *Mini golf?*

Who would enjoy doing these with you?

How can you reduce the junk food at your next holiday?

For example:

- *Replace Halloween candy with stickers?*
- *Play more games and eat fewer courses?*
- *String cranberries and popcorn instead of baking holiday cookies?*

Whom should you talk to about making this happen?

CHAPTER 15

Struggling with

Emotional

Eating?

The toughest part of emotional
eating for many clients is the self-
blame that comes from *knowing
better* while they do it. A good
coach helps clients redirect this
frustration into practical strategies
to:

- Prevent negative emotions,
  when possible, and

- Find healthier ways to deal with emotions, rather than overeat.

Because emotions can be powerful and sneaky, I like to guide clients to self-experiment and to embrace the idea of gradual improvement via trial and error.

These questions get you started.

Which emotions tend to make you eat?

For how long does the emotional eating make you feel better?

Which specific situations tend to make you eat emotionally?

Can you prevent these situations? If not, how can you handle them smarter?

How frequent and extreme are your feelings of loneliness, sadness, anxiety, etc.?

Do you need any professional help managing these emotions?

What activities make you feel happy and relaxed, without eating?

Can you schedule some of these activities *right now*?

Are there ways to prevent some of your negative emotions?

For example:

- *Make more social plans to prevent loneliness?*
- *Learn a new hobby to prevent boredom?*
- *Be more organized to prevent stress?*

What specific preventative steps could you take now?

If you are bored, what are 10 things you could do besides eat?

For example:

- *Call a friend?*
- *Browse new apps?*
- *Play with a pet?*

What items should you have ready, so that it's easy to do these smarter activities?

If you are lonely, what are 10 things you could do besides eat?

For example:

- *Join an online forum?*
- *Attend an exercise class?*
- *Call a friend?*
- *Write a letter?*

What items should you have ready, so that it's easy to do the right thing?

If you are anxious, what are 10 things could you do besides eat?

For example:

- *Call a friend?*
- *Take a bath?*
- *Stretch?*

What items should you have ready, so that it's easy to do the right thing?

If you are frustrated, what are 10 things you could do besides eat?

For example:

- *Clean a closet?*
- *Do a set of push ups?*
- *Chop veggies for future meals?*

What items should you have ready, so that it's easy to do the right thing?

If you are seeking pleasure, what are 10 things you could do besides eat?

For example:

- *Get a facial?*
- *Take a warm bath?*
- *Trade foot massages?*

What items should you have ready, so that it's easy to do the right thing?

What are 10 ways to celebrate happy events without overeating?

For example:

- *Small gifts?*
- *Dancing?*
- *Decorations?*

What can you plan or prepare *right now* to make your next celebration healthier?

CHAPTER 16

Struggling with
Everything?!

When absolutely everything feels difficult, there is a good chance that a client is feeling generally overwhelmed, stressed or exhausted...from working at her nutrition program or anything else in life. Addressing these underlying issues can often reduce the feeling of struggle. Or, maybe the client just needs a shot of inspiration. Or more realistic goals. Finding and addressing the problem is your job as a good coach!

These questions get you started.

Are you well-rested?

If not, how can you get there?

Are you overwhelmed by other pressures or priorities?

Is this temporary or a normal state of being? How can you make time and energy for your health?

Have you had your yearly physical?

Should you consult your doctor about whether you have issues with thyroid, hormones, depression, or anything else?

What was different when you last had success at this?

For example:

- *Your diet?*
- *Your sleep?*
- *Your work schedule?*
- *Your routine?*
- *Your social group?*

Can you recreate those old successful conditions?

What small healthy things *can* you do, even if they seem insignificant?

For example:

- *Drink 8 cups water?*
- *Walk the dog?*

Can you stick to these for 1 week?

Who gets you inspired?

How can you spend some time with them?

Would you be better off thinking *less* about this?

What if you "just do it" for a week, and see if habits start to solidify?

Is eating your main pleasure in life right now?

How can you get more varied pleasures into your life?

CHAPTER 17

Ready for the
Ever-After?

A good coach teaches her clients to:

- Regularly assess how things are going
- Foresee and prevent potential problems
- Recognize common threats, like a change in routine
- Recognize danger signs, like prolonged fatigue and stress
- Plan for relapse.

When clients are empowered with a smart game plan for the ever-after, they can confidently enjoy their new bodies, rather than live in fear of another yo-yo cycle.

These questions get you started.

Which healthy habits are going well?

Can you keep it up?

Which health habits are not going well?

Why? What would it take to improve them?

Are there any healthy opportunities on the horizon?

For example:

- *Kids getting old enough to help with cooking?*
- *New fun exercise class being offered?*
- *Summer bringing tastier fresh produce?*

How can you best take advantage of these opportunities?

Do you see any possible threats on the horizon?

For example:

- *Holidays bringing temptations?*
- *Less time for yourself because of schedule changes?*
- *Eating out for a month while kitchen is remodeled?*

What is your game plan for handling these threats?

What upcoming life events might break your normal routine?

For example:

- *Getting married?*
- *Having a child?*
- *Changing jobs?*
- *Traveling?*

How will you establish a new healthy routine ASAP?

When life throws you off track, what will you do?

Are you comfortable knowing that when relapse happens, you can always rebuild another successful routine, based on your new circumstances?